Stiff

with M

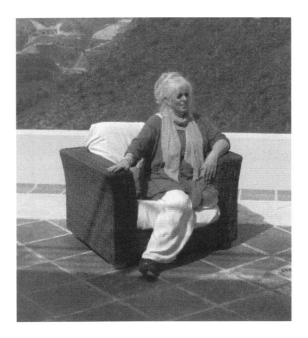

Can you get up groan free from your armchair?

Do you avoid getting down on your knees because you need major scaffolding to get you back up?

Stiff and aching joints can lurk behind the corner for us all. Be it caused by arthritis, uric acid, fibromyalgia or just 'wear and tear'.

Let Madison share some practical self-help techniques, based on diet, energy medicine and common sense. They stand by themselves or support any treatment you may be receiving.

Published in Great Britain

All paper used in the printing of this book has been made from wood grown in managed, sustainable forests.

ISBN13: 978-1-78003-618-2

Essential Book Series

First published by Indepenpress Publishing Limited

25 Eastern Place

Brighton

BN2 1GJ

For Author Essentials

A catalogue record of this book is available from

the British Library

Cover design © Author Essentials

info@authoressentials.com

Stiff joints – CONTENTS

Two one liners from my past often pop into my mind and make me laugh:

Victoria Wood once said: *"You know you're getting old when you walk past Dr Scholl's and think 'Hmm, they look COMFY'."*

Well, I did just that the other day when I walked past a shoe shop and even worse, I have now become enamoured with elastic waistbands, and the cosiness, on Winter nights, of my pink fleecy dressing gown: come on own up, I am not alone in this am I? Please tell me that you feel the same sometimes!

Do some of you feel as if you are standing at the foothills of 'old age' not particularly well equipped to clamber up and enjoy the heights?

Billy Connolly said:*"You know you're getting old when every time you get up from the armchair you grunt or groan!"* Horror of horrors, a grunt like groan escaped my lips the other day when I got up from my sofa which seems to have become strangely lower over the past few months.

None of us are immune to stiff, aching or arthritic joints especially in the morning. What can be done to help relieve that pain?

First of all, let's look at what can cause inflexible articulations:

What is arthritis?

It is actually a generic term that covers various conditions, including the four listed below. It has always existed but our modern lifestyles, with increased stress and toxic overload, contribute to the 'stiffness epidemic' in the Western world.

Osteo arthritis.

This degenerative joint disease is the most common form of arthritis. Weight bearing joints such as the knees, hips and spine are particularly vulnerable. In a nutshell; the cartilage covering the bones and surrounding the joint wears away. The smooth surfaces become rough and eventually, in severe cases, bone will literally rub on bone causing extreme pain.

Normally it can start in our 40s [although rules like this always invite exceptions] and emerges gradually over the years. It is more common in women than men and can 'run in families'. Be suspicious of any joint with lessened mobility and a 'grating' or 'clicking' sound or sensation when moved.

Rheumatoid arthritis – RA.

This is a chronic, auto-immune, inflammatory disease predominantly affecting the synovial membrane lining the joint. When it becomes inflamed it damages and destroys adjoining tissue, causing stiffness and pain. It greatly restricts the use of the joint. It is quite literally a 'self-attacking' condition.

RA generally has an earlier onset age of 25-50 and while osteoarthritis will affect specific joints, RA can affect all the body's synovial joints.

As one would expect, synovial joints are characterised by the presence of synovial fluid within the joint. Each synovial capsule reduces the friction between the bones, allowing for a smoother movement. They are the most common joints in the body and include: elbow, knee, hip, thumb etc.

In addition, with RA secondary problems can arise, including:

- Digestive troubles

- Fatigue

- Colitis

- Lung and bronchial congestion

- Liver problems

- Inflammation of the blood vessels

- Inflammation of the outer lining of the heart and lungs

Common contributory causes include:

- Calcium depletion

- Hormone imbalance

- Prolonged use of aspirin or cortico-steroid drugs

- Poor diet [i.e. processed, refined, chemical rich foods]

Rheumatism.

Excessive uric acid settles in the joints causing them to inflame. Improving your body chemistry and nurturing your Liver, with careful attention to diet and detoxification can help relieve this condition.

Gout.

A metabolic disorder featuring excessive uric acid [I'll talk more about uric acid later in this booklet] resulting in sudden swelling and pain in the hands, knees or toe joints. The classic being the big toe. Working with some of the techniques in this booklet may help.

I would also mention injury, either past or present. It may be that as a child you fell down, bounced up again and never thought anything of it, but perhaps you slightly damaged the bone or connective tissue and over decades that slight damage began to cause real mischief in your body's symmetry and function.

I always encourage people, when their children fall down, to take them to a doctor, cranio sacral osteopath, physiotherapist — whoever they have confidence in locally and get the child checked out. A little attention at that early stage can perhaps save years of stiffness later on in life.

So these are the key contributors to stiff joints and painful movement. What I would like to achieve with this booklet is for you to try out, with objective assessment, the techniques that 'read right' to you. It is impossible to do everything, so be discerning and choose what you feel might help. Do it and then sit quietly and tune into your body:

- Has it helped?

- Do you feel an improvement?

- Did you enjoy doing the technique?

- What do you 'feel'?

If the answers are all positive, then continue with that technique in your daily life. If not, try another. The important thing is to keep trying until you find the key that unlocks the door to a definite improvement in your symptoms.

Be sensible and if you have the slightest whisper of concern, consult your healthcare practitioner before doing anything. RA especially is very sensitive to changes in your life, in whatever sense be it diet or exercise.

WHAT CAN YOU DO?

WATCH YOUR WEIGHT

Weight can indeed be a key factor in either causing or aggravating pain or stiffness, particularly in the back, hips and knees. Losing just a few pounds can make all the difference to the comfort and flexibility of your movements.

It is said that every extra pound of weight on your body feels like 4lbs pressure on your knees. It is commonsense that we should each lose our excess pounds. This is my area of 'challenge' as I love my grub and know when I go past a certain weight it is like turning on a switch to pain. Equally when I go below that weight pain and discomfort lessen considerably with the reduced load.

So, I would advise you to consider losing those extra pounds, in whatever way suits you. I am a huge fan of Weight Watchers and I find that gone are the days of cardboard crisp breads and calorie counting; WW have become a very healthy way of eating.

I would advise strongly against any diet that is extreme.

Use commonsense.

I am well qualified to write this booklet. I have test driven most of what I have suggested and everything has helped, to a lesser or greater extent, control my pain and stiffness. I do believe we have predisposition to arthritis, my mother and every one of her sisters have been crippled by the most appalling arthritic pain.

I also believe we can talk ourselves into it. We get what we expect. So don't programme yourself into stiffness, expecting to get it just because your mother did. Yes, you might have a tendency to it, but there is LOTS you can do to stop it or reduce it. Don't give in; remain optimistic and positive about your ability to remain flexible.

pH balance

Try to improve your **acid/alkaline balance** – most of us are far too 'acidic' and discomfort and pain can be lessened by a more alkaline body environment.

This can be achieved primarily through changes to your diet. Try cutting out the following foods and see how your joints react. Eliminate them all, or, if that is too daunting a prospect, eliminate one by one, observing your body's reaction, the proof of the pudding is in how *you feel*... it may not be just your joints that feel better, you may have more energy, be more optimistic/positive, be less bloated, skin may improve etc.,

Foods to avoid if you wish to achieve a healthier acid/alkaline balance include:

6

- *Sugar, refined, convenience and processed foods* – let's not beat about the bush,sugar is an addictive 'drug' and like many of the 'ingredients' in refined, processed or convenience foods can cause chemical chaos in our bodies. Be cautious with anything 'white'.

- *Excessively fatty/fried foods* – although a little olive oil is excellent, a deep friend battered chocolate bar is not!

- *Dairy products* – if this is difficult for you to eliminate, experiment with Goat or sheep cheese/Soya milk – persevere, you will develop a taste for them. They are far easier for the body to digest.

- *Wheat* – substitute with Ryvita original, rye or spelt bread. Organic where possible

- *Excessive salt* – read labels so that you are aware of 'hidden' salt

- *Fizzy drinks* – again some are highly addictive and you will have to wean yourself off them, but worth the effort. Try an alternative such as sparkling water mixed with a little apple or cranberry juice [sugar free of course].

- *Chocolate* – if that is a bridge too far try this: buy really good quality, organic high % chocolate, put in the fridge and break yourself off one big square a day, smell it, taste it and suck it to make it last longer – that is your daily fix. Far better one square than a whole bar.

- *Coffee* – if you find it too hard to give up, cut down and only drink good quality beans – no instant or decaffeinated, both often contain chemicals.

- *Tobacco* – no lectures, you know the risks

- *Alcohol* – moderation is the keyword

Finally, take a deep breath or two – it alkalises the body.

EATING FOR ENERGY

Your first port of call should be to experiment with eliminating the above foods and observe how your body reacts. However, if you are interested in Kinesiology and energy testing, let me share a simple self testing technique whereby you can actually have a dialogue with your body to see what foods strengthen in at this moment in time and what foods stress it. Naturally, if you keep your eating habits to foods that your body finds easy to process, there is less build up of acid and pain can lessen.

There are many self testing techniques but I would like to focus on one in particular that most people find easy and reliable. You will be using your body as a pendulum:

- stand, barefoot if possible,

- feet solidly on the floor, not too far apart,

- knees unlocked,

- take a deep breath,

- set the intention that you want an honest dialogue with yourself, that you seek the truth, you seek knowledge. What you do with that knowledge once you have it is entirely your choice.

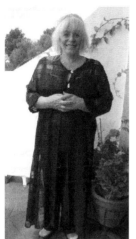

Place one hand over your solar plexus and the other hand over the first.

Tuck your elbows into your sides.

Close your eyes and say *"my name is Minnie Mouse"*. Now, does your body sway forward or backward?

Repeat the test but this time saying *"my name is [your name]"* – what happens?

Normally the body will sway forward toward the truth or a substance that is strong/ positive and easily metabolised and backward i.e. away from one that is weak/negative, does not suit the body chemistry, or an untruth.

It will either be attracted or repelled. You will sway forward or backward.

However, rules are always made to be broken and some people buck this trend. You may even vary occasionally. By using the Minnie Mouse test you can establish your personal weak and strong sway for that day.

WITH FOODS: simply hold the sample against the solar plexus or navel and see in which direction you sway. Normally a forward sway indicates your body will tolerate that food and a backward sway that it is better to eliminate the food from your diet, at least for ten days and observe how you feel.

As you can see, it takes a little time and discipline but over the coming weeks you can identify, through self testing, experiment and observation, what works for you. Once you have this information you can adapt your lifestyle accordingly and you will realise it is all well worth the effort as you begin to note improvements.

URIC ACID

It is worth saying something about uric acid as it can contribute to pain, especially gout. We all have uric acid; it's a waste product from the normal process of cells dying and releasing purines. The body also absorbs purines from some foods.

In a healthy body, uric acid is dissolved in the blood and passes, through the kidneys, into the urine and eliminated. Problems begin when more uric acid is produced than the kidneys can deal with.

If uric acid levels reach an abnormally high level, they can form sodium urate crystals in the joints. Your doctor can measure your uric acid levels through a simple blood test – ideally you should have a level of less than 6.0mg/dl.

Don't ignore a high uric acid level – discuss the matter with your doctor – there are various diets that can help lower the level. Primarily reducing purine rich foods in your diet. Foods that contain high purine levels include:

- meats such as liver

- shellfish

- eggs

- yeast

- tomatoes

- cheese

- tuna

- salmon

- sardines

- turkey

- pulses/lentils

- cherries

- berries

- rhubarb

- acidic food

- juices

- vinegar

- alcohol

- bacon

- trout

In addition, because of the kidney connection – Trace your kidney meridian daily to help strengthen it and increase its efficiency. Your hands are like electromagnetic pads and when you align them with the energy flows, the energy will follow the hands, it will move and in tracing, it will move along the pathways and increase efficiency of the related organ, in this case the Kidney.

> Place your fingers under the ball of each foot, on the line where the colour changes – middle finger in line with the space between your first and second toes; draw your fingers up to the inside of each foot, circle behind the inside of each ankle bone, and go straight up the front of the body to K27, the points beneath the clavicle at the top of the sternum; vigorously press and rub these points.

THE WONDER OF WATER

If we hydrate the body, it can regenerate and

heal itself beyond our wildest imagination.

Alkalise your water. Search on Amazon for pH test strips that can be used with either urine or saliva to see if you are an acid drop or an alkaline angel.

There are also drops that can be added to your water to alkalise it and therefore help achieve a healthy pH balance in your body.

However, no point doing it unless you are acidic – so test first to see if there is a need. [visit Alkalive www. ph-ion.com].

They say that future wars will be fought over this precious commodity that we, in the Western world, take so much for granted. Who knows? But we do know that, more than food, water truly is the essence of life, a vital energy source and without which we will die.

Do not deceive yourself, the majority of us are seriously dehydrated and we don't even know it, as symptoms are easily misdiagnosed.

Increase your water consumption and watch your overall health improve, lower backache vanish, heartburn, migraine and hunger pangs diminish, fibromyalgia pains lessen, asthma and allergies reduce and daytime fatigue disappear. As the brain is 85% water, water is indeed 'food for thought' that can help all aspects of brain alertness and function.

Are you drinking enough? If your urine is mid- dark yellow, probably not. Experts recommend 6–8 [1½–2 litres] per day. The sensation of thirst is not triggered until you are *already* dehydrated, so drink BEFORE you get thirsty. Increase your intake of fresh fruit and veg as they have high water content. However, tea, coffee and sodas rob the body of water. There is no substitute for water, it helps:

- The body metabolise fat
- Suppress the appetite, so is an aid to losing weight
- Prevent DNA damage
- Prevent constipation
- Keep joints mobile
- Keep skin soft and subtle – cheaper than La Praire!
- Prevent slack and sagging skin after weight loss
- Prevent premature ageing
- Production of vital hormones and amino acids

- Keep arteries clear
- Generate electrical and magnetic energy inside each cell – it is 'power' food
- Convert food into energy
- Remove toxins from all parts of the body
- Maintain a healthy acid alkaline balance – drinking water should ideally be a little alkaline with a pH level of 7.5
- The body stay cool
- Strengthen the immune system and fight colds and other viruses

Many people say they can't drink more water as the increased urination can interfere with everyday life! But compare it to watering a dried out pot plant, at first the water will rush right through, after a few days or weeks of careful watering, the water will be more easily absorbed and the rush will be lessened. Once the body learns to absorb the increased water intake, urine flow will become normal.

Another concern can be water 'retention'. The body retains water because it fears dehydration. In most cases, give it what it needs, take away the fear and it will release stored water.

According to Dr Batmanghelidj [Water & Salt – your healers from within] *'every 24 hours the body recycles the equivalent of 40,000 glasses of water to maintain its normal physiological functions'*. It runs short of about 6-8 glasses a day and these are what need replacing. Ideally water should be drunk:–

- 30 minutes before eating,

- 2½ hours after a meal,

- whenever you are thirsty,

- first thing in the morning,

- before exercising

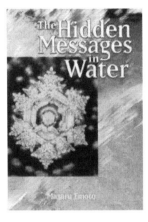

Obvious you might say, what is she going on about but THINK, what was your water drinking pattern in the past 24 hours?

Water can store and transmit information. Dr Masaru Emoto [The Hidden Messages in Water] claims that if human speech or thoughts are directed at water droplets before they are frozen, images of the resulting water crystals will be beautiful or ugly and chaotic depending upon whether the words or thoughts were positive or negative.

This can be achieved through prayer, music or by attaching written words to a container of water. The most powerful words emerged as LOVE and GRATITUDE. Tape these words to your bottle of water to positively energise it. I have made little laminated mats with love and gratitude printed on them and my water stands on this as does my animal food and my food!

If you read his book it has compelling photographic evidence of the positive change in water molecules. Just think, our bodies are 75% water, so will be affected in the same way as the glass of water!

Another way to revitalize water is to use crystals such as amethyst, clear, smoky or rose quartz. Place the crystal in a jug, filter jug, or even in your dog's water bowl [make sure the crystal is large enough so that the dog cannot swallow it] or for the green fingered, the watering can. Leave for 8 hours then use.

Magnetising water can help regenerate it into a more healthy state of vitality. It can help:

- prevent cholesterol from depositing in blood vessels,

- improve digestion

- enhance the blood supply and nutrition to various organs.

Place a glass jug of water on top of the _north_ side of a large magnet and leave for 10 minutes–24 hours. If you can't identify north from south, one simple solution is to tape the north pole of a magnet onto one side of a glass jug of water and the south pole on the other side... you don't even have to know exactly which is which, just remember opposites attract.

If you can find a 'lipstick' shaped magnet [used to remove metallic debris from cattle feed] stir the liquid with the magnet.

If you have no magnets to hand simply use your own magnetism – hold slightly cupped hands opposite each other, an inch away from the sides of the glass. Stay in this position for a minute then drink the water.

Magnetised water can be stored in a fridge for up to ten days.

If, like me, you find water a tad boring and a full glass a bit of a challenge, why not:

- have your very own water bottle and take sips throughout the day,before you know it, you will have emptied the bottle.

- Add a slice of lemon or lime, a dash of organic cordial [okay, so it ceases to be 'pure' water, but if it means you drink more, it is worth the 'pollution']. In the summer make a strong dilution of organic herbal fruit tea, keep it in the fridge as an alternative 'cordial'.

The final question has to be WHAT SORT OF WATER? The ideal is natural spring water, not many of us have one of those in our back gardens, and we simply use bottled water [preferably glass and never leave a plastic bottle of water in the sun, the warmth encourages chemicals in the plastic to leach into the water]. Failing that, tap water through a filter is a good option.

Looking at the state of an electric kettle after a few days of use may put you off using plain tap water, the calcium deposits in our bodies particularly our veins, in the same way.

Sadly carbonated is not as good as 'still' water for our health, but IS better than coffee!

So, crack open a bottle, pour a glass, sit down, relax, drink it slowly. Tell yourself that this water is hydrating every single cell of your body, eliminating toxins and bringing you health and vitality – that is the wonder of water.

Apple Cider Vinegar, organic honey and hot water – an excellent way to start the day. You might think it is too acidic but it is actually alkalising.

Oil the joints withFlaxseed/**Linseed oil** [they are the same] – can easily be taken in capsule form.

Glucosamine Sulphate is a popular supplement to help reduce pain. It is involved in the formation of bones, cartilage and joint fluid [synovial]

If there is inflammation try **Quercetin/Bromelain** capsules. You can take them orally and also make up a poultice to place over the joint. Open up 3-4 capsules and mix with a few drops of pure olive oil and spread over the area – cover with a little cling film then muslin and put your leg up and watch your favourite TV programme.

I am hearing great reports on **turmeric** capsules. It has been used in India for centuries. It is one thing I have not yet tried, but I am about to. I certainly use a lot in cooking, also known as Indian Saffron.

I have personally used **Magnesium Oil spray** – the trans dermal delivery gets the magnesium to where it is needed straight away.

Other supplements that might interest you:

- Nettle tisane can help counter arthritis

- Cat's Claw tea for pain relief

- Siberian ginseng is especially beneficial for rheumatoid arthritis

- Selenium an anti-oxidant needed to repair free radical damage

- Barley grass is particularly good for gout

- Spirulina is anti-inflammatory and can protect joints against destruction

- Linseed or Split Hempseeds – I sprinkle mine [about a tablespoonful] onto salads, muesli etc.,

- Silica – helps rebuild connective tissue

- Vitamin E can increase jont mobility

- Zinc picolinate is often deficient in arthritis sufferers

- CoQ10 repairs connective tissue

- B Complex for the nervous system

- Black Molasses is a rich source of the B complex vitamins, iron, copper and magnesium

- Feverfew helps reduce pain

- Folic Acid, if you suffer RA you might be deficient

Naturally you will not take them all. I recommend you try one supplement at a time and observe how it affects your body. Another good investment of your time and money is to find a local reputable nutritionist and some health stores have experienced staff who are qualified to provide useful advice.

FLOWER ESSENCES

Oh the world is indeed your oyster, there are so many flower essences easily available now. Perhaps my favourite brand is the Australian Bush Flower Remedies www.ausflowers.com.au

The ones that stand out for me include:

Sturt Desert Pea – can help release old sorrow and/or grief

Black Eyed Susan – if you only ever bought one essence, buy this one, great for stress.

Southern Cross – victim mentality, bitter, martyrs

Yellow Cowslip Orchid – critical, judgemental or nit picking – rigidity

Dagger Hakea – resentment, bitterness, forgiveness

Hibbertia – inflexibility, dogmatic, in control, rigidity of the mind

Little Flannel Flower – brings spontaneity and lightness [often lacking if you suffer physical stiffness or pain].

Other little anti-stiffness tips

Get out in the **sunshine**, when there is some, as it helps the production of Vitamin D, which is involved in bone formation.

Magnets

Magnets are an effective way to help relieve arthritic pain. Simply lay the **north** side of a small magnet against your pain. Tape it onto the site and leave for an hour. Needless to say, don't go near a magnet if you have a pacemaker or any metal in your body.

A number of people find comfort wearing copper bracelets. You could try one and see if it helps.

How to find the north side of a magnet.

There is huge confusion over magnet polarity as different countries call them different names. A simple way to identify polarity is to energy test.

Hold one side of the magnet against your left ear and energy test a strong indicator muscle (e.g. deltoid). If you are not familiar with energy testing – visit You Tube and there are various clips demonstrating how to do it.

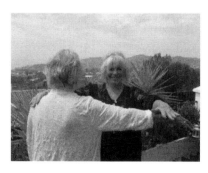

- Your friend stands up straight, un-clenched and relaxed, with feet apart. [If necessary, the test can be done sitting].

- Left arm [or right] is held out at a right angle to the body and parallel to the floor – this isolates the muscle, see position in photo.

- Check hand is *not* clenched into a fist – fingers should be straight.

- Stand in front of your friend, not too close, with your right hand, palm flat and facing downwards and fingers extended – resting on your friend's raised arm, on the forearm near the wrist joint. [Shoulder side of the wrist].

- The left hand can rest gently on her shoulder.

- Demonstrate the range of movement – so that she is confident in what is about to happen. *You are interested in the first couple of inches* of that range, not everyone's arm drops all the way down to their hip. It might be that a 'spongy' response is all that is felt, but that is enough to indicate a weak result.

- Tell her to 'HOLD' – wait half a second, while her brain registers the command and then apply pressure for 2 seconds – gently, no jerking movements.

- What happened? If it locks and stays in position easily it means that it is testing STRONG.

- However, if it is spongy, or falls all the way down then that is a WEAK test.

If it is the first time testing, it is a good idea to check that the person is testing correctly. You do this by the following procedure:

Weaken them by running the palm of your hand backwards along the Central meridian[1] [down the centre of their torso].

TEST – it should be weak i.e. the arm will go down or be spongy. Now run your palm up along the flow of Central [up the centre of the torso].

TEST – it should be strong.

This gives you a feel of their individual range and confirms they are testing correctly.

To find the North side of the magnet, hold it against your head, just above your ear.

Now test

If you are **STRONG** the side against your head is **SOUTH** (it actually disperses the energy to your extremities)

It can also be called 'north seeking'.

If the test is **WEAK** the side against your head is **NORTH** (it is pulling energy away from your extremities)

It can also be called 'south seeking'.

Do not depend upon the commercial labelling of magnets.

---

1 Tracing backwards on any channel of energy will weaken the body. Central runs up the body, so tracing down the body is against the flow and will weaken the person. At the end of the test, always ensure you trace upwards to leave the person strong.

Bigger is not necessarily better as far as magnets are concerned. Start with small round ones.

Incidentally, if no tape is available, two flat magnets, one worn inside and one outside clothing can be used to treat a specific area... the magnetism keeps them in place.

First identify the north and south polarities as demonstrated in the above test.

THE NORTH SIDE (south seeking)

- Sedates and calms energy

- Contracts

- Stabilises

- Balances

- Restful and restorative

It can therefore be used to

- Take away pain

- Reduce swellings

- Combat infections

- Lower blood pressure

- Inhibit tumour growth

- **Help sprains, broken bones,**

- **Arthritis, toothache etc.,**

Spiral out the pain

A truly ancient self healing technique that is simple, easy and quick is to use your hands to lift out the pain. Or have a loved one do it for you.

Hold a clear quartz crystal in your hand as you spiral [optional].

Before you start, take some deep breaths, focus, concentrate and briskly rub the palms of your hands together and the 'shake them off' to get rid of any stagnant energy that may have accumulated in your hands.

- Place your left hand gently on or over the painful joint.

- Circle that hand in an anti-clockwise direction for a few minutes. Slowly moving it further away from the body.

- Imagine you are drawing out stagnant, negative or toxic energies from the body.

- Rub your hands together, shake off any excess 'energy' you may have drawn out of the site.

- Place your right hand gently on or over the painful joint

- Slowly circle this hand in a clockwise direction for a couple of minutes. You are now harmonising, strengthening and balancing that area's energy, which helps reduce pain.

- Rub your hands together, shaking them off

- Trace a figure 8 over the area for a few seconds.

Tapping away pain

A hairbrush is not just for the hair, learn how your plastic Denman can help reduce stiffness and pain in the body

One of the fundamental beliefs of energy medicine is that wherever there is pain in the body, there will also be 'stagnation' of some kind: blood, lymph, energy, nerve connections – nothing will be flowing or operating smoothly. Energy becomes 'stuck' and can even begin to move backwards along the meridians, causing toxic build up. This, combined with years of wear, tear and probable abuse, results in stiffness and pain, especially in the joints, back, neck and shoulders.

One technique to get things moving is simply to 'hairbrush tap' – it will be as if 100 little fingers are stimulating the area:–

- Buy a hairbrush, the style with hard plastic 'spikes'

- With a light wrist, gently tap all over the joint area with the spiky side of the hairbrush. It should feel as if you are bouncing the spikes off your body.

- Tapping can be in any direction, speed or pattern you wish.

- The area should be covered with material – it can be irritating to tap directly onto skin.

- Tap for 10 seconds or 10 minutes – whatever feels good or is convenient.

- Rub, in an anticlockwise circle, over the painful area with either the heel of the hand or with the fingers. An anticlockwise direction tends to 'lift' pain out of an area.

You may like to use some oil to help the process – a few drops of the essential oils Black Pepper and Sweet Marjoram diluted in a carrier such as Sweet Almond Oil, smell divine as they warm and relax the area. Creams that contain Wintergreen, menthol, eucalyptus, camphor etc., are useful tools in your arsenal against rigidity and pain.

- To finish, 'brush off' the limb with the flat palms of your hands. For example, if you were tapping the knee joint you would end by placing both palms on either side of the knee and with a light pressure, slide the hands down to the feet and come off the toes.

- End by tracing Figure 8s [Tibetan healing symbol of infinity] over the area.

It is inexpensive and takes very little time or effort. Many of my clients over the years have used this deceptively simple technique and have experienced fantastic results: return of sensation in an area, reduced pain, increased movement etc., My teacher and friend Donna Eden tapped away her MS [sounds remarkable? Google her or read her book Energy Medicine for the full story]

Keep the brush in eyesight, maybe by the bed, television, computer – wherever you will *see* it. That way it will remind you to tap. If it is stuck away in a draw, believe me, you will forget to do it!

Tibetan Figure 8

In Tibetan Medicine, the **figure 8** shape is well respected for its healing properties – with your fingers, trace the shape over the painful joint, almost like doodling – do it 5 minutes at a time, when you are watching television or reading. It doesn't matter if it is a horizontal or vertical 8, big or small, just trace what feels right to you.

Stretching

Stretching is vital to retain as much flexibility as possible. It also creates space for toxins to exit joints, where they might be accumulating and causing mischief.

Stretches should be slow, never jerky. Never force anything into the arena of pain. If you can only move 1 inch and not 1 foot – it's ok, it is the stretch that counts, not the distance.

Consider joining a stretch class, Alexander Technique or Feldenkrais and of course, yoga – look around in your area; often it is the teacher that will sway you.

Practice intuitive stretching; experiment with simple moves that create space in your body, especially in the spine. Let go of your inhibitions and move into the realms of flexibility.

Crystals

OK, this might be outside your realm of knowledge or even comfort but crystals have been used for healing for many centuries in many different cultures. The absolute worst they can do is nothing, so why not try them – small tumbled crystals are relatively inexpensive and easy to find.

www.charliesrockshop.com or www.rockngem.co.uk/show

If you live in London the above shop and event are well worth visiting.

Crystals that offer pain relief include:

- **Malachite** – calms the painful area, draws out imbalances and absorbs negativity. Raises the spirits and increases hope.

- **Green Calcite** – aids release of old rigid belief systems, transition from stagnation to movement. Stimulates the immune system. Very good for arthritis, bone adjustments and problems with the ligaments and muscles.

- **Turquoise** – calm, healing energy. Stimulates the immune system and meridians. Good all round protection and strengthening.

- **Carnelian** – encourages healing of any damaged tissue

- **Rose Quartz** – promotes inner peace and forgiveness

- **Clear Quartz** – brings harmony and strengthens energy

- **Amethyst** – versatile all purpose healer

- **Black Tourmaline** – specifically good for muscular and skeletal problems

Select one that you feel resonates with you, that you are drawn to.

It can be used in many ways:

- Hold it against the painful joint for a few minutes

- Using micro tape, attach it to the painful area for an hour or so a couple of times a day or when particularly painful.

- Simply hold it in your hand, rolling it around and feeling it with all your senses.

- Sleep with it under your pillow

- Hold it while you do figure 8's over the joint

- Hold it while circling over the joint

- Wear in the form of jewellery

- Carry it in a pouch in your pocket or around your neck

A specific technique is to use a clear quartz crystal to 'pull out' pain.

- Circle above the pain in an anticlockwise direction for 20 seconds or so; moving further and further away from the body.

- Cleanse the crystal under running cold water.

- Circle clockwise over the pain with the crystal.

- [or invest in two crystals then you can cut out the cleaning in between]

- End with figure 8ing for ten seconds over the area. It disperses the density of energy in a painful area; dense energy is always present where there is pain.

Another technique to disperse dense energy and pain is to gently figure 8 **Selenite** above the area for a minute or two. According to the School of Crystal Acupuncture[2] this is an excellent technique to do before massaging as it helps clear the energy and therefore increasing the ability to get deeper into the muscle tissue.

LARGE INTESTINE 4

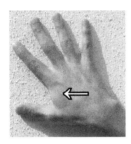

This is the fourth acupressure point on the flow of energy called large intestine – which naturally relates to digestion but is also an important point for relieving pain in general. It is said to be anti inflammatory too. This point is used a lot with athletes and knee injuries.

The official description for finding the point is: *On the dorsum of the hand, between the first and second metacarpal bones, approximately in the middle of the second metacarpal bone on the radial side.*

A cheat's way of find it is to squeeze the thumb against the index finger hard and a 'hump' emerges, on the top of that lump is the point. Once located hold the point or squeeze the lump firmly for 30 seconds, relax and repeat.

2 The crystal therapy training school Wales
website www.visionforliving.co.uk
email kimdowdell@visionforliving.co.uk

A word of caution though, never use this point if you are pregnant it can promote a miscarriage or labour.

GALLBLADDER 31

This point is located on the outside thigh, between the knee and hip. If you stand with your shoulders and arms relaxed, the middle finger will automatically fall on this point.

Massage firmly for a few seconds, relax and repeat.

RUB WOOD

The entire traditional Chinese health system is based on the 5 element philosophy, created after centuries of observation and discernment. In this tradition, it is believed that Wood element governs flexibility and therefore, if we experience any stiffness in our bodies, we should look to the health [both physically and energetically] of the Liver and Gallbladder meridians of energy. One of the simplest ways of doing this is to massage the reflex points associated with both these organs, it encourages release of toxic waste and a balancing of the energies, which reflects in the physical.

LIVER is the easier to locate, it lies under the right underwire in your bra. Lift up your breast and massage, very firmly, along the line where the bra sat. Just a few seconds will be enough on a daily basis.

GALLBLADDER – on either side of your lower sternum [breastbone] massage from bottom to half way up – firmly.

SPINAL FLUSH

Taking this lymphatic massage further, consider a spinal flush:

We are all familiar with the body's lymphatic system; garbage disposal at its best, key to our immunity, helping counter conditions ranging from colds to cancer.

The lymphatic system is bigger than the circulatory system, but does not have a heart to pump the lymph around the body; it relies on gravity and exercise/movement. With our increasingly sedentary lifestyles, the system can become sluggish and less effective in clearing toxins from certain parts of the body. When this happens the 'garbage' can accumulate and cause very real problems.

To maintain a healthy lymphatic system: move, walk, body brush, drink water, get a regular massage and do a daily 'Spinal Flush'.

"What is a Spinal Flush?" I hear you ask.

It is simply a firm massage along either side of the spine. Through clothes or directly on skin, it stimulates certain 'neurolymphatic reflex points' that trigger the garbage disposal system into activity and encourage the efficient removal of toxins from the body and strengthen immunity.

You will feel more energized and optimistic as the body begins to rid itself of stagnant energies and emotional residue.

It also stimulates the cerebrospinal fluid, clearing your head.

If you feel the very first signs of a cold coming on, a Spinal Flush can stimulate your immunity enough to nip it in the bud.

In fact, if you did this every day to each other, you may not even catch a cold in the first place!

It is a great technique for partners as it quickly dissolves built up stress and takes the edge off any 'emotional overreaction' [an understated way of saying things getting a little heated and you are about to either become a foulmouthed fishwife, go into a tight lipped sulk or flounce out the door!]. So, rather than head towards an argument and divorce proceedings, give each other a spinal flush, an inexpensive form of marriage counselling without words!

If any of the points feel sore, unless there is an obvious reason, such as a bruise, injury or medical condition, the soreness indicates that the point, and its corresponding organ, need a bit of attention, so linger on the point a little longer. However, if you are recovering from an illness or suffer an autoimmune problem, you may find a lot of the points are sore. If this is the case, go easy so as not to overwhelm the system.

To do the Spinal Flush takes about a minute, but is so enjoyable you may well be pleading 'don't stop!'.

Lie face down, or stand 2-3 feet from a wall and lean into it with your hands supporting you at chest level, or above your head as in the photograph. This positions your body to remain stable while your partner applies pressure to your back.

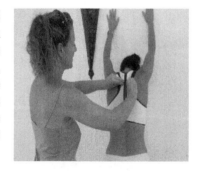

Your partner massages the points down either side of your spine, using the thumbs, fingers or knuckles and applying body weight to get strong pressure but no rough, jerky or sudden movements.

Massage from the bottom of the neck all the way down to the bottom of the sacrum. Go down the notches between the vertebrae and deeply massage each point for a few seconds, moving the skin in a circular motion with strong pressure but ensuring that the pressure is comfortable.

This technique should not feel painful. Make sure neither of you are holding your breath.

Upon reach your sacrum, your partner can repeat the massage or complete it by 'sweeping' the energies down your body, from your shoulders, and with an open hand, all the way down your legs and off your feet, 2-3 times.

Each of these points relate to a specific energy meridian/ organ but do not be concerned about what they are, just work down the spine, giving a little extra time and attention to any that 'sore'.

If you dwell a bit on the points just above the sacrum, they relate to Bladder which governs 'fear' which is an emotion that often stops us stepping out with courage and doing what our heart wants to do.

I suppose I should say, please use your common sense and do not do a Spinal Flush if there is even a whisper of spinal injury, bruising or problems in the area. If in any doubt check with your healthcare practitioner.

Okay, so what happens if you don't have a willing partner? Then, two tennis balls in a sock are going to be your best friends!

Place two tennis balls in a sock and tie the end tightly. Lie on your back with knees bent and feet flat on the floor. Raise your body up slightly and place the balls under the top of the spine. The spine itself will sit comfortably between each ball. Pressure should never be applied directly to the bone itself, but to the muscles on either side of the spine. Lower your weight on to the ball and wriggle around so it massages the neurolymphatic reflex points.

Alternatively, you can just lie on top of the balls and after about 30 seconds you will begin to feel the back relax and the points 'opening'. Do this down the entire length of the spine, spending a little extra time on any sore spots.

If getting up and down from the floor is not easy for you, an excellent variation [in fact it is my favourite] is to place the balls on a wall, ideally on a corner, or door jam. Feet should be placed about 18" away from the wall [the further away the more pressure is applied to the back]. Lean your full body weight against the balls. Bend knees to manoeuvre them up and down the spine, wriggle around and pay attention to the sore points. Sit against the balls on a plane, it helps reduce back pain, you might get a few funny looks but your back will benefit.

There is another technique with these tennis balls that you might like to try:

Place them under the head so the weight of the head rests on the balls.

Ideally positioned in a small indentation your will find half way up the skull, on the centre line.

If you don't have the tennis balls you can rest your head

on your two clasped fists, but make sure it is not causing tension in your muscles.

This reduces stress and fear in the body. If it feels a bit too strong for you, just use the palm of your hand.

LOTIONS AND POTIONS

1. **Arnica or an essential oil**, blended into a warm carrier oil such a Sweet Almond, and gently, rhythmically and slowly massaged onto the inflamed or painful area can bring some relief. Essential oils to consider are: Benzoin, Lavender, Myrrh, Sweet Marjoram, Juniper, Black Pepper, Vetiver, Yarrow, Ginger and Rosemary. Touch is a powerful healer. Focus your intention on 'love' and 'healing' when you massage yourself or a friend and remember the spirally and Figure 8 techniques.

2. **MSM** cream by Higher Nature, has biologically active sulphur.

3. Good old fashioned **Wintergreen** is still available. As with all these stronger oils/creams – be careful with your eyes. Obviously don't apply it to any sensitive area and take care, after you have massaged to wash your hands, otherwise you rub your eyes a few minutes later and boy it stings!

4. **Comfrey** cream – in ancient times Comfrey was known as 'knitbone' because of its power in the healing of broken bones. Search in the local health stores or go online.

    Alternatively, why not grow your own comfrey and make a tincture to rub on the joints.

It is said that if you soak your feet in a bowl of comfrey infused water, the healing properties will enter and circulate your body via the soles of your feet.

5. **Aloe Vera** gel [keep it in the fridge and apply if joints become hot and swollen, particularly calming in the Summer heat]. Ice can be soothing – use frozen peas rather than ice itself, it has the advantage of being more 'flexible'. Never apply ice or peas directly to the skin, put a cloth in between, to prevent 'burning'.

6. **Cooling balms** that contain camphor, menthol, Eucalyptus. Tiger Balm is a favourite. If you go to London pop into one of the Chinese Herbalists, they stock some great medicated balms a particular favourite of mine is WONG TO YICK WOODLOCK – I kid you not!

7. **Epsom Salt** bath – take a long, hot bath with a mugful of Epsom Salts mixed in. The salts have the ability to draw out toxins from the body/joints and the warmth of the bath is relaxing. Add a few drops of lavender essential oil before you step in. Shower off afterwards and then rub joints with one of the creams mentioned above.

USE IT IF YOU CAN

The problem with painful stiff joints is that we are naturally reluctant to use them, consequently our range of movement slowly reduces over time and suddenly we find that it is less than 50% and decreasing annually. **Gently move/stretch** the joints every day, use them, don't let the boundaries close in. Check your **posture**, could it be improved? Is it compensating for pain and creating more problems?

The emotions of stiffness

Is the stiffness in your body reflecting stiffness in your thoughts or attitudes?

Are you being a little too judgemental/critical of others or even yourself?

Could you benefit from being a little more flexible, lightening up slightly?

Are you plagued by 'toxic' thoughts, frustration, resentment, anger and other assorted negative emotions?

Take a few minutes to sit and contemplate this aspect of your life. Be honest with yourself and then work on letting go of the emotions of stiffness.

DON'T GET THE HUMP!

Have you noticed the small fatty padded 'knuckle' that can stealthily appear at the very top of the back/neck area, as we age? Often called a Buffalo or Dowager's[3] Hump its medical term is Kyphosis and in advanced cases results in a bent-over posture. Kyphosis is a result of advanced osteoporosis, the vertebrae of the spine become so porous that they can weaken and often fracture.

However, I am more interested, in this booklet, on focussing on the *beginning* of a hump, to see if there

---

3 'Dignified older lady' is the definition of Dowager, which I think is rather charming.

is anything we can do to avoid its appearance in our lives.

The key is posture: it is essential to keep the spine straight and in correct alignment, all day, every day. The Alexander Technique is excellent to re educate the body and gently encourage it away from bad postural habits. If you don't have a therapist or teacher locally what can you do yourself?

Strengthen the abdominal girdle so that the back is not having to do work it was not designed to do. Check your posture right now. No, don't straighten up, how are you _really_ sitting, what is the cold honest truth? Are you a true couch potato; slumped in the chair, tummy relaxed and protruding, back curved, neck bent and head thrown back as you focus through your glasses?

Here is a simple exercise and one you can do anywhere, anytime; in fact do it RIGHT NOW – suck your navel right in, try and get it to touch your spine [remember in the 60s when we squeezed ourselves into tight jeans, lying on the floor with a coat hanger in the zip, slowly zipping it closed? Well, that's the feeling; breathing your tummy in as far as it will go to get into a pair of tight trousers]. Release it 50% and stay with that for as long as you can. In reality that is how our abdominal girdle should be engaged all the time. You might not believe me, but if you could get that girdle working efficiently myriad back problems would magically disappear as the abdominal muscles do the job they were designed to do and the back can stop troubleshooting. In addition, with improved posture the organs have more room in which to function. The ultimate benefit of course, is you will immediately look slimmer and younger! _I call this technique TUMMY TUCKING for this reason._

> Put up sticky notes everywhere with 'TT'
> written on them and every time you see one
> – tummy tuck!

Another easy technique:

- Place the heel of your right hand on your forehead with your fingers curled over your head.

- Note where your middle finger lands and imagine a thin silver cord stretching from this precise point up to the sky.

- The cord tightens and pulls you up off your heels.

- Stay there for a second and then gently lower the heels keeping the head and neck in position.

- Ensure you are 'tummy tucking', breathing normally and smiling.

- Remove the hand from above the head and with the middle finger gently push the chin in/back towards the spine, only a tiny amount; this will have the effect of further correcting the position of the neck.

- You are probably sitting or standing there feeling a little odd in this position but it is the posture you should be aiming for all the time.

Look for a Pilates class near you, it is an excellent way to strengthen your abdominal girdle.

As I keep saying, stagnation is the friend of pain but your enemy. So keep everything moving in the neck and upper back by exercise, stretching, massage and hairbrush tapping.

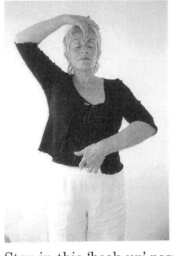

Do a little self-reflexology and firmly massage all around the base of the big toe, down and around the bunion joint.

Do the Hook Up – place the middle finger of the right hand in the navel and the middle finger of the left hand on the 3rd eye in the space between your eyebrows. Close your eyes, breathe deeply, press in with both fingers and gently pull up. Stay in this 'hook up' position for 20 seconds as it will encourage the flow of energy up the spine. If energy flows through an area, flexibility improves.

Bones are associated with Water Element which governs 'fear' in our lives; what are you fearful of? Confront it, pick it to pieces in your mind, it is often not as bad as we imagine. Let go of the fear and start believing that 'all will be well'.

Yoga is a gentle yet effective way to spinal health.

- Try looking over the left shoulder as far as you can, keeping the girdle engaged and posture correct.

- Repeat on the right hand side.

- Return your head to the centre and lower your right ear to your right shoulder [don't cheat and lift the shoulder].

- Repeat on the left side.

Hold all these movements for a minimum of 10 seconds.

- End by letting the head fall forward and slowly rolling it around to the left, back to centre and then around to the right, returning to centre. Lift it up slowly.

[never, ever throw your head straight back, it can result in injury].

Obviously do not attempt any form of neck exercise if you are injured in that area, always check with your Doctor first.

Finally, when I was a schoolgirl we were made to walk around the classroom with a book balanced on our heads – sounds very Victorian doesn't it but you know, they had some pretty good ideas. Try it right now and watch your posture instantly improve – think of how straight and upright native women can appear when carrying bundles on their heads. Try and get up out of the chair and walk around the room with the book balancing. When you are sitting at the computer, keep a book on your head to prevent you slipping down into damaging posture.

Do not feel helpless – there are a lot of things you can try to relieve the pain and discomfort of stiff joints. Read through this little booklet and decide what appeals to you and try it, give it enough time to have an impact. We live in a society that encourages the 'instant fix' – sometimes things take a little longer to work.

Look on the bright side of life; be positive, flexible in thought and attitude. Stretch, move, swim, walk. Watch your diet and pH balance. Lose some excess weight. Experiment with lotions, potions and crystals. Try some of the energy medicine techniques and watch your posture [both standing and sitting].

Observe objectively the results; you may not be able to totally eliminate pain, but you may be able to reduce it to a more acceptable level.

---oOo---

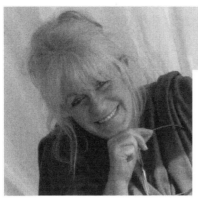

MADISON KING
writer and teacher of energy medicine

Madison's Medicine is a unique fusion of energy and body work, flower essences, lifestyle advice and commonsense – providing essential, everyday, practical tools for a healthier and happier you.

Many moons ago Madison was involved in the heart of London advertising, becoming a successful international board director. However, she realised, after a few ambition fuelled years, that she wanted her life to take a different direction and shocked everyone by giving up the BMW, Armani suits and Gucci briefcase, becoming a student again.

She trained in massage, sports massage, aromatherapy, Indian head massage, reflexology, trager, nutrition, flower essences, crystals, radionics... A true workshop groupie, she filled a wall with qualifications but could not find what she had been seeking; she couldn't even really define it... until, through divine synchronicity, she met Donna Eden in London through a mutual friend. Within no time at all she was in Ashland in Donna's backyard with about four other students, eagerly learning about energy – this was more than two decades ago, so no information highway was available in those days and ever the thirsty student she drank in everything she could on these visits, rushing back to London to experiment on her long suffering clients!

Over the years she crossed the ocean many times learning from Donna and also John Thie [Touch for Health].

She then began to teach Donna's work in the UK, USA, Gozo, Malta, Italy, Egypt and many other locations around the world, she has appeared on national television, radio and press promoting EEM. She haslectured at Westminster and Oxford universities and at the key Mind Body Spirit Festivals in London and Wales.

In 2006 she gave up a thriving practice in Central London and now divides her time between the Isle of Wight and the Andalucían town of Nerja in Southern Spain.

Just about to enter her 7th decade, she has set up and is running Donna Eden's training in Europe – based just outside London... a long way from those days in Donna's back yard!

Her focus is on promoting Donna's work in Europe and also writing and teaching her own version: Madison's Medicine, which based on Eden Energy Medicine also weaves in many other natural health threads, giving people simple yet powerful tools to enhance their quality of life on every single level.

As we enter unprecedented waters on this planet, it can be empowering to know that there is always something YOU can do to improve any situation, challenge or trauma that life throws into your path.

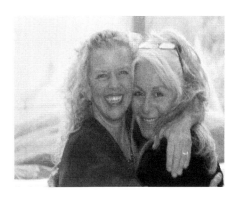

"*Madison is an extraordinary woman and healer. She carries an essence of the highest quality and caring, of camaraderie of spirit, wisdom, compassion and depth of understanding of the healing realms. To train with her is something you will never regret*"

Donna Eden – Eden Energy Medicine

Madison can be contacted:

www.madisonking.com
www.midlifegoddess.ning.com
madisonking@hotmail.com

My special thanks to Donna Eden.[4]

Without her friendship and generous, unselfish sharing of her vast knowledge, I would not be who I am today and you would not be reading this book.

If this whets your appetite for more information on books, DVD, CDs online study and workshops visit

www.midlifegoddess.ning.com

and also Donna Eden's site, I strongly recommend her book Energy Medicine

www.innersource.net

You Tube for some great clips

And look out for other books in the Essentials stable

---

4 www.innersource.net